Surviving Prostate Cancer

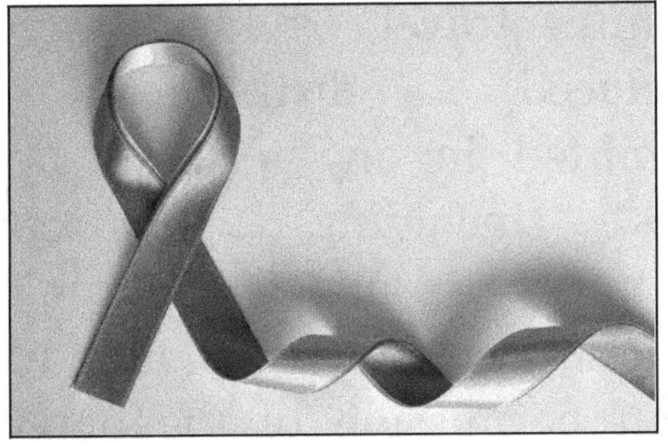

A Guide to Early Detection, Treatment, and Recovery.

Grace Parker

Table of Content

Introduction

Importance of prostate cancer awareness and prevention

Prostate cancer is a disease that affects the male reproductive system and is the most common cancer in men after skin cancer. It is estimated that one in eight men will be diagnosed with prostate cancer in their lifetime, making it a serious health concern for men. Although it is a serious disease, prostate cancer can often be detected and treated successfully, especially if detected early. In this book, we will discuss the importance of prostate cancer awareness and prevention.

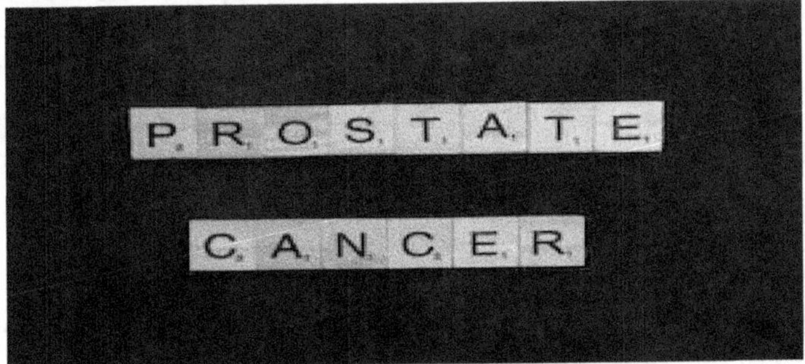

One of the main reasons why prostate cancer is such a significant health concern is that it often does not produce any symptoms in its early stages. This means that men can have prostate cancer without even knowing it. However, as the cancer grows and progresses, symptoms such as difficulty urinating, blood in the urine or semen, and pain in the back or hips may appear. Unfortunately, by the time these symptoms appear, the cancer may have already spread beyond the prostate gland, making it more difficult to treat.

The key to dealing with prostate cancer is early detection. This is where prostate cancer awareness and prevention come in. Men need to be aware of the risk factors associated with prostate cancer, including age, family history, and ethnicity, and should take proactive steps to reduce their risk. This includes getting regular prostate cancer screenings, which are typically recommended for men over the age of 50 or men with a family history of prostate cancer, and adopting a healthy lifestyle, such as a balanced diet, exercise, and stress management.

Prostate cancer awareness and prevention can also play a significant role in reducing the number of deaths caused by this disease. According to the American Cancer Society, the 5-year survival rate for prostate cancer that has not spread outside of the prostate is nearly 100%. However, this drops to just 30% for prostate cancer that has spread to other parts of the body. This result highlights the significance of early detection and treatment.

In conclusion, prostate cancer is a serious health concern for men, but it can often be detected and treated successfully if caught early. Prostate cancer awareness and prevention are essential in reducing the number of advanced cases and improving survival rates. Men should be aware of the risk factors associated with prostate cancer, get regular screenings, and adopt a healthy lifestyle to reduce their risk. By raising awareness and promoting prevention, we can make significant strides in the fight against prostate cancer.

Understanding prostate cancer and its risk factors

Prostate cancer is a type of cancer that develops in the prostate gland, which is a small, walnut-shaped gland that is part of the male reproductive system. The prostate gland is situated just below the bladder and in front of the rectum. The primary function of the prostate gland is to produce and secrete the fluid that makes up a part of semen.

The exact cause of prostate cancer is not known, but there are several risk factors associated with the disease. Some of the most common risk factors for prostate cancer include:

Age: Prostate cancer is more common in older men, and the risk increases as men get older. In fact, about 60% of prostate cancer cases are diagnosed in men over the age of 65.

Family history: Men with a family history of prostate cancer, especially a father or brother who had the disease, are at higher risk of developing prostate cancer themselves.

Ethnicity: Prostate cancer is more familiar in African American men than in men of other ethnicities. Additionally, men of Caribbean descent and men with a family history of prostate cancer are also at increased risk.

Diet: There is some evidence to suggest that a diet high in red meat and high-fat dairy products may increase the risk of prostate cancer.

Genetic mutations: Inherited mutations of certain genes, such as BRCA1 and BRCA2, have been linked to an increased risk of prostate cancer.

Inflammation: Chronic inflammation of the prostate gland, often caused by an infection, has been associated with an increased risk of prostate cancer.

Hormonal imbalances: High levels of certain hormones, such as testosterone, may increase the risk of developing prostate cancer.

Environmental exposures: Exposure to certain environmental factors, such as pesticides, may increase the risk of developing prostate cancer.

Medications: Some studies have suggested that certain medications, such as statins or aspirin, may reduce the risk of prostate cancer, while others, such as nonsteroidal anti-inflammatory drugs (NSAIDs), may increase the risk.
Lifestyle factors: Obesity, lack of exercise, and smoking have all been linked to an increased risk of prostate cancer.

It is crucial to note that having one or more of these risk characteristics does not necessarily mean that a man will have prostate cancer. Likewise, not having any risk factors does not guarantee that a man will not develop the disease. However, by understanding the risk factors associated with prostate cancer, men can take steps to reduce their risk and increase the chances of early detection.

In addition to understanding the risk factors associated with prostate cancer, it is important for men to be aware of the signs and symptoms of the disease. Some common symptoms of prostate cancer include difficulty urinating, weak or interrupted urine flow, the need to urinate frequently (especially at night), blood in the urine or semen, and pain or discomfort in the pelvic area. Men who experience any of these symptoms should see a doctor promptly to determine the cause and receive appropriate treatment.

In conclusion, understanding the risk factors associated with prostate cancer is an essential part of prevention and early detection. By knowing the risk factors and being aware of the signs and symptoms of the disease, men can take steps to reduce their risk, receive timely diagnosis and treatment, and improve their chances of survival.

Chapter 1

Diagnosis and Staging

Symptoms of prostate cancer

Prostate cancer is often detected through routine screening tests, such as a digital rectal exam (DRE) or a prostate-specific antigen (PSA) blood test. During a DRE, a healthcare provider inserts a lubricated, gloved finger into the rectum to feel for any abnormalities in the prostate gland. A PSA test measures the level of a protein called prostate-specific antigen in the blood. High PSA levels may indicate the presence of prostate cancer.

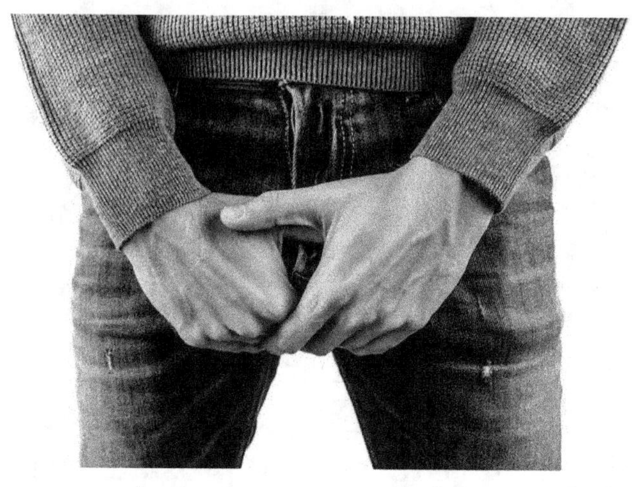

If a screening test suggests the possibility of prostate cancer, a healthcare provider may order additional tests to confirm the diagnosis and determine the stage of the cancer. Some common diagnostic tests for prostate cancer include:

Biopsy: During a biopsy, a healthcare provider removes a small sample of prostate tissue and examines it under a microscope for the presence of cancer cells.

Imaging tests: Imaging tests, such as a CT scan, MRI, or bone scan, may be used to determine the extent of the cancer and whether it has spread to other parts of the body.

Once a diagnosis of prostate cancer has been confirmed, it is important to determine the stage of cancer. Staging is a process that helps to determine how far cancer has spread and to develop an appropriate treatment plan. The most commonly used staging system for prostate cancer is the TNM system, which stands for Tumor, Node, and Metastasis. This system describes the size of the tumor (T), whether the cancer has spread to nearby lymph nodes (N), and whether the cancer has metastasized or spread to other parts of the body (M).

Symptoms of prostate cancer can vary from person to person, and some men may experience no symptoms at all. However, it is important for men to be aware of the potential symptoms of prostate cancer so that they can seek medical attention if they experience any of these signs.

One of the most common symptoms of prostate cancer is difficulty urinating or a weak urine flow. This may be due to the fact that the prostate gland surrounds the urethra, which is the tube that carries urine from the bladder out of the body. As the cancer grows, it may cause the prostate gland to enlarge, which can put pressure on the urethra and make it more difficult to urinate.

Another common symptom of prostate cancer is frequent urination, especially at night. This is also due to the pressure that the growing cancer places on the urethra, which can cause the bladder to become overactive and increase the urge to urinate.

Blood in the urine or semen may also be a symptom of prostate cancer. This occurs when the cancer cells invade the blood vessels in the prostate gland, causing them to rupture and release blood into the urine or semen. While this may be alarming, it is important to note that blood in the urine or semen may also be caused by other medical conditions, such as an infection or inflammation.

Pain or discomfort in the pelvic area may also be a symptom of prostate cancer. This may occur as the cancer grows and puts pressure on the surrounding tissues and organs, causing pain or discomfort. In advanced cases of prostate cancer, the cancer may spread to other parts of the body, such as the bones, which can cause bone pain or fractures.

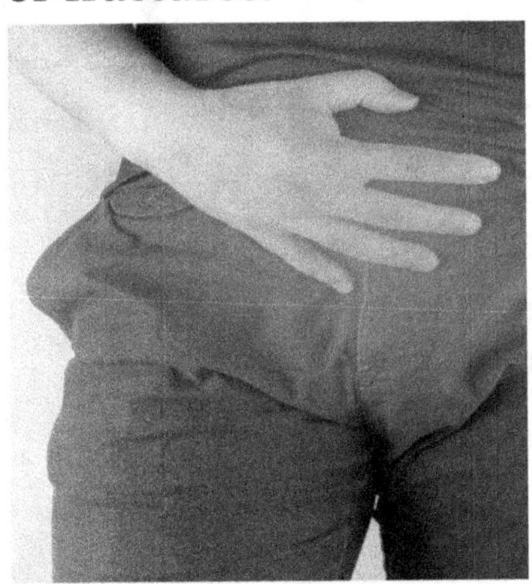

Painful ejaculation: Prostate cancer may cause pain or discomfort during ejaculation. This is because the cancer may invade the nerves that control ejaculation or cause inflammation in the prostate gland.

Swelling in the legs or feet: Advanced prostate cancer that has spread to the lymph nodes may cause swelling in the legs or feet. This is because the lymph nodes in the groin area, which drain fluid from the legs, may become blocked by the cancer.

Loss of appetite or weight loss: Prostate cancer may cause a loss of appetite or unintended weight loss. This is because the cancer may release chemicals that affect the way the body uses energy, or it may interfere with the digestive system.

Fatigue: Prostate cancer may cause fatigue or a general feeling of weakness. This is because the cancer may use up the body's energy or cause the body to produce less red blood cells, which carry oxygen to the muscles.

In addition to these symptoms, prostate cancer may also cause erectile dysfunction, which is the inability to achieve or maintain an erection. This may be due to the fact that the nerves that control erectile function run close to the prostate gland, and damage to these nerves during cancer treatment may cause erectile dysfunction.

It is important to note that these symptoms may also be caused by other medical conditions, and not all men with prostate cancer will experience symptoms. However, men who experience any of these symptoms should see a healthcare provider promptly to determine the cause and receive appropriate treatment. Early detection and treatment of prostate cancer can improve outcomes and increase the chances of a full recovery.

Prostate cancer screening and diagnosis

Prostate cancer screening and diagnosis are important for early detection and treatment. The screening process involves testing for prostate cancer in men who do not have any symptoms of the disease. The diagnosis process involves further testing for men who have symptoms or who have received an abnormal result from a screening test.

There are two major tests used for prostate cancer screening:

Prostate-specific antigen (PSA) test: This is a blood test that estimates the level of PSA, a protein secreted by the prostate gland. A high level of PSA in the blood may indicate the presence of prostate cancer or other prostate conditions. However, a high PSA level does not always mean that a man has prostate cancer, and a low PSA level does not always mean that a man does not have prostate cancer.

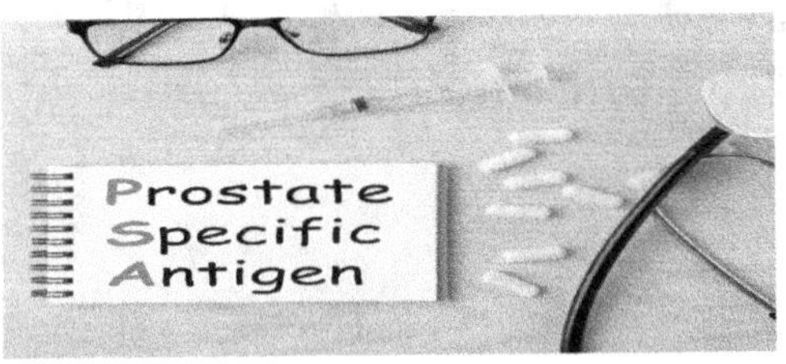

Digital rectal exam (DRE): This is a physical exam in which a healthcare provider inserts a gloved, lubricated finger into the rectum to feel the prostate gland for any abnormalities, such as lumps or hard spots. The DRE may be used in combination with the PSA test to screen for prostate cancer.

If the screening tests suggest the possibility of prostate cancer, further tests may be needed to confirm the diagnosis, such as:

Biopsy: This is a procedure in which a small sample of prostate tissue is removed and examined under a microscope to look for the presence of cancer cells. A biopsy may be recommended if the PSA level is high or if a lump or other abnormality is found during the DRE.

Imaging tests: These tests, such as ultrasound, MRI, or CT scan, use high-frequency sound waves or magnetic fields to create detailed images of the prostate gland and surrounding tissues. These tests may be used to help determine the size and location of the cancer, as well as whether it has spread to other parts of the body.

It is important to note that not all prostate cancers require immediate treatment, and some may not require treatment at all. The decision to treat prostate cancer depends on a variety of factors, including the stage of the cancer, the man's age and overall health, and the potential benefits and risks of treatment. Men who are at risk for prostate cancer or who have symptoms should talk to their healthcare provider about the benefits and risks of screening and the best approach for their individual situation.

Staging of prostate cancer

Staging is the process of determining how far cancer has spread in the body. For prostate cancer, staging is based on several factors, including the size and location of the tumor, whether it has spread to nearby lymph nodes, and whether it has spread to other parts of the body. The most commonly used staging system for prostate cancer is the TNM system, which stands for Tumor, Nodes, and Metastasis.

The T category of the TNM system describes the size and location of the primary tumor:

T1: The tumor is not palpable (can't be felt) and is only found through imaging tests or biopsy.

T2: The tumor is confined to the prostate gland and can be felt during a digital rectal exam.

T3: The tumor has grown outside the prostate gland and may have invaded nearby tissues or organs, such as the seminal vesicles.

T4: The tumor has spread to nearby structures, such as the bladder or rectum.

The N category describes whether the cancer has spread to nearby lymph nodes:

N0: The cancer has not circulated to nearby lymph nodes.

N1: The cancer has circulated to nearby lymph nodes.

The M category describes whether the cancer has circulated to other parts of the body:

M0: The cancer has not circulated to other parts of the body.

M1: The cancer has spread to other parts of the body, such as the bones, liver, or lungs.

Using the TNM system, prostate cancer is typically staged from I to IV, with higher stages indicating more advanced disease. For example, early-stage prostate cancer may be classified as T1 or T2N0M0, while advanced-stage prostate cancer may be classified as T4N1M1.

Staging is an important part of determining the appropriate treatment for prostate cancer. Treatment options may include surgery, radiation therapy, hormone therapy, or a combination of these treatments. Men with prostate cancer should talk to their healthcare provider about the stage of their cancer and the best treatment options for their individual situation.

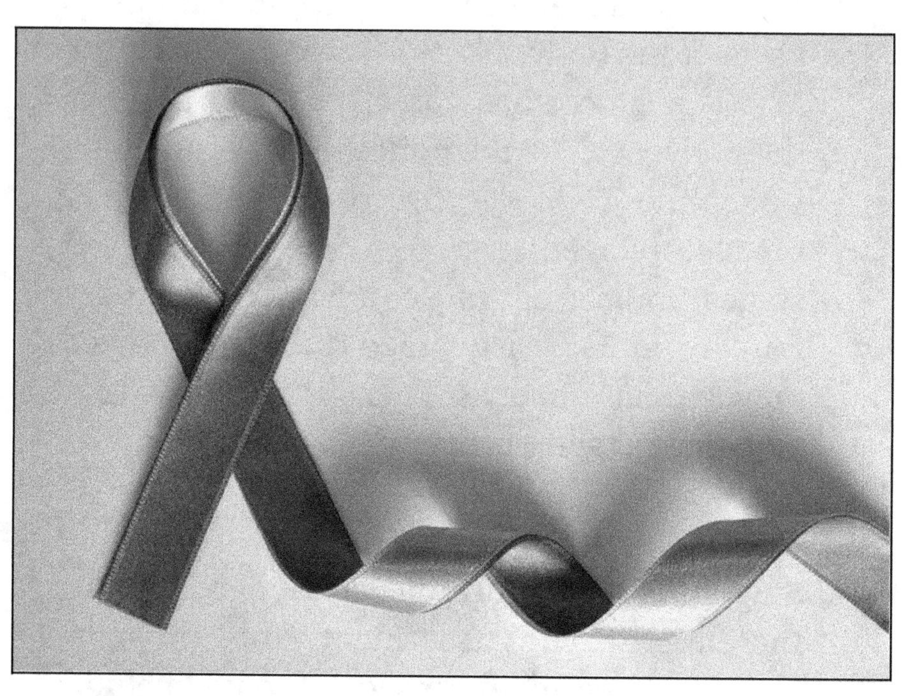

Chapter 2

Treatment options

Active surveillance

Active surveillance, also known as watchful waiting, is a treatment option for men with low-risk prostate cancer. Active surveillance involves monitoring the cancer closely over time with regular check-ups, blood tests, and biopsies, but not treating it immediately. This approach is based on the understanding that many prostate cancers grow very slowly and may never cause significant problems during a man's lifetime. Active surveillance allows men to avoid the potential side effects of treatment, such as impotence and incontinence, while still providing the opportunity to start treatment if the cancer shows signs of progressing.

Active surveillance may be recommended for men who have a low-risk prostate cancer, which means the cancer is small, confined to the prostate gland, and growing slowly. The criteria for low-risk prostate cancer may vary, but typically include:

- A PSA status of less than 10 ng/mL
- A Gleason score of 6 or less
- A tumor that is confined to one part of the prostate gland.

Men who choose active surveillance will need to have regular check-ups with their healthcare provider to monitor their cancer. This may include:

PSA tests: Blood tests to measure the level of prostate-specific antigen (PSA) in the blood. PSA levels may be used to monitor the growth of the cancer over time.

Digital rectal exams (DRE): Physical exams to feel the prostate gland for any changes or abnormalities.

Imaging tests: Tests, such as ultrasound or MRI, to create detailed images of the prostate gland and surrounding tissues.

Biopsies: If there are any signs of the cancer growing or changing, a biopsy may be performed to remove a small sample of prostate tissue for examination under a microscope.

If the cancer shows signs of progressing, such as an increase in PSA levels or changes in the biopsy results, treatment may be recommended. Treatment options for prostate cancer may include surgery, radiation therapy, hormone therapy, or a combination of these treatments.

Active surveillance is not appropriate for all men with prostate cancer. Men who have high-risk prostate cancer, which means the cancer is more aggressive and more likely to spread, may not be good candidates for active surveillance. Men who are considering active surveillance should talk to their healthcare provider about the benefits and risks of this approach and whether it is appropriate for their individual situation.

Surgery

Surgery is a common treatment option for prostate cancer. The goal of surgery is to remove the entire prostate gland and any cancer that may have spread outside of the gland. The most common type of surgery for prostate cancer is radical prostatectomy, which is the removal of the entire prostate gland, along with the seminal vesicles and nearby lymph nodes.

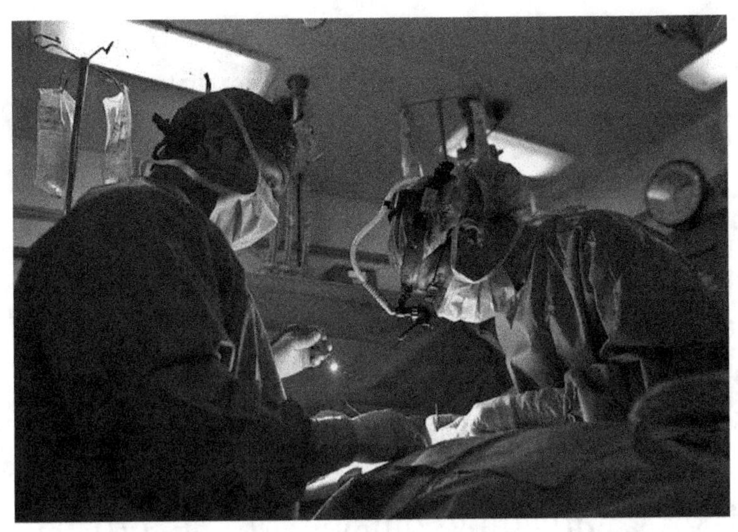

Radical prostatectomy can be performed using different approaches, including:

Open surgery: The surgeon makes a large incision in the abdomen to access the prostate gland and surrounding tissues.
Laparoscopic surgery: The surgeon makes several small incisions in the abdomen and uses a camera and specialized instruments to remove the prostate gland.

Robot-assisted laparoscopic surgery: The surgeon uses a robotic system to control the surgical instruments and perform the surgery through small incisions in the abdomen.

Surgery may be recommended for men with early stage prostate cancer, especially if the cancer is confined to the prostate gland and has not spread to other parts of the body. Surgery may also be recommended for men with localized prostate cancer that is at high risk of spreading outside of the prostate gland. In some cases, surgery may be combined with other treatments, such as radiation therapy or hormone therapy, to improve the chances of a cure.

Surgery carries the risk of side effects, including:

Erectile dysfunction: Surgery may damage the nerves that control erection, resulting in difficulty achieving or maintaining an erection.

Incontinence: Surgery may damage the muscles and nerves that control urination, resulting in difficulty controlling urine.

Blood loss: Surgery may result in significant blood loss, which may require a blood transfusion.

Infection: Surgery may increase the risk of infection at the surgical site or in other parts of the body.

Men who are considering surgery for prostate cancer should talk to their healthcare provider about the benefits and risks of the procedure, as well as the potential for side effects. They should also discuss their risk factors for side effects and how to manage them after surgery.

Radiation therapy

Radiation therapy is a common treatment option for prostate cancer. It uses high-energy radiation, such as X-rays or protons, to destroy cancer cells and shrink tumors. Radiation therapy can be provided externally or internally.

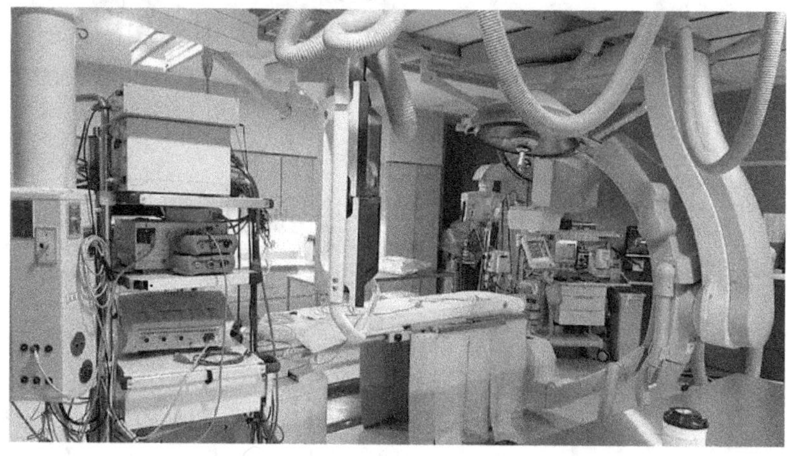

External beam radiation therapy involves directing a beam of radiation at the prostate gland from outside the body. This is typically done using a machine called a linear accelerator, which delivers a high dose of radiation to the prostate gland while minimizing exposure to surrounding healthy tissues. External beam radiation therapy may be given daily over several weeks, with each treatment session lasting only a few minutes.

Internal radiation therapy, also known as brachytherapy, involves placing small radioactive seeds directly into the prostate gland. The seeds give off radiation to destroy the cancer cells over time. Brachytherapy is typically performed as an outpatient procedure and may be used alone or in combination with external beam radiation therapy.

Radiation therapy may be recommended for men with early-stage prostate cancer or for men with advanced prostate cancer that has spread to other parts of the body. It may also be used after surgery to destroy any hanging around cancer cells.

Radiation therapy carries the risk of side effects, including:

Urinary problems: Radiation therapy may irritate the bladder and urethra, resulting in urinary frequency, urgency, and discomfort. Rectal problems: Radiation therapy may irritate the rectum, resulting in diarrhea, bleeding, and discomfort.

Erectile dysfunction: Radiation therapy may damage the nerves and blood vessels that control erection, resulting in difficulty achieving or maintaining an erection.

Fatigue: Radiation therapy may cause fatigue and low energy levels.

Skin changes: Radiation therapy may cause redness, irritation, and dryness of the skin in the treated area.

Men who are considering radiation therapy for prostate cancer should talk to their healthcare provider about the benefits and risks of the treatment, as well as the potential for side effects. They should also discuss their risk factors for side effects and how to manage them during and after treatment.

Hormone therapy

Hormone therapy, also known as androgen deprivation therapy (ADT), is a treatment option for prostate cancer that works by reducing the levels of male hormones, such as testosterone, in the body. Prostate cancer cells depend on these hormones to grow and spread, so by reducing their levels, hormone therapy can help slow down or stop the growth of the cancer.

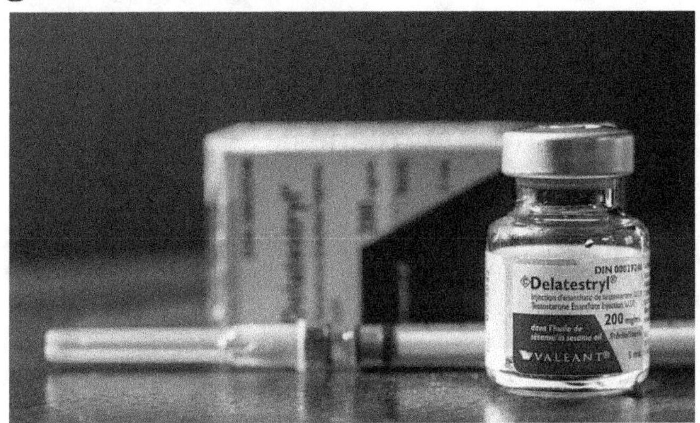

Hormone therapy can be delivered in several ways, including:

Medications: Hormone therapy medications are taken orally or injected into the body. They work by blocking the production or action of male hormones in the body.
Surgery: In some cases, the testicles may be surgically removed to reduce the production of male hormones.

Hormone therapy may be recommended for men with advanced prostate cancer or for men with early-stage prostate cancer who are at high risk of recurrence. It may also be used in combination with other treatments, such as radiation therapy or chemotherapy, to improve their effectiveness.

Hormone therapy carries the risk of side effects, including:

Loss of libido: Hormone therapy may reduce sexual desire and performance.

Erectile dysfunction: Hormone therapy may interfere with the ability to achieve or maintain an erection.

Hot flashes: Hormone therapy may cause sudden and intense feelings of heat and sweating.

Fatigue: Hormone therapy may cause fatigue and low energy levels.

Osteoporosis: Hormone therapy may increase the risk of bone loss and fractures.

Men who are considering hormone therapy for prostate cancer should talk to their healthcare provider about the benefits and risks of the treatment, as well as the potential for side effects. They should also discuss their individual risk factors for side effects and how to manage them during and after treatment.

Chemotherapy

Chemotherapy is a treatment option for prostate cancer that uses drugs to kill cancer cells. Unlike radiation therapy or surgery, which targets the cancer cells in a specific area of the body, chemotherapy works throughout the body and may be used to treat cancer that has spread to other parts of the body.

Chemotherapy is typically given through a vein, either as an injection or through an IV (intravenous) line. The drugs are then carried through the bloodstream to reach the cancer cells. Chemotherapy may be given in cycles, with a period of treatment followed by a period of rest, to allow the body to recover.

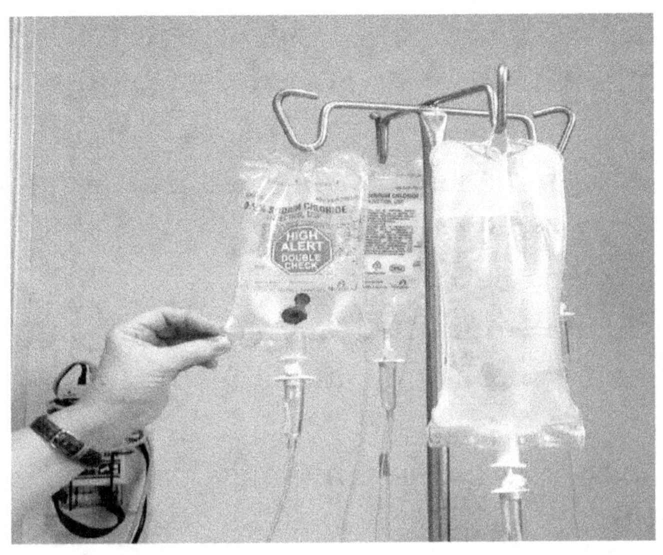

Chemotherapy may be recommended for men with advanced prostate cancer that has spread to other parts of the body, or for men who have not responded to hormone therapy. It may also be used in combination with other treatments, such as radiation therapy or surgery, to improve their effectiveness.

Chemotherapy carries the risk of side effects, which can vary depending on the drugs used and the individual's response to treatment. Common side effects of chemotherapy for prostate cancer include:

Fatigue: Chemotherapy may cause fatigue and low energy levels.

Nausea and vomiting: Chemotherapy may cause nausea, vomiting, and appetite loss.

Hair loss: Chemotherapy may cause hair loss or thinning.

Mouth sores: Chemotherapy may cause sores in the mouth or throat.

Increased risk of infection: Chemotherapy may reduce the number of white blood cells in the body, increasing the risk of infection.

Men who are considering chemotherapy for prostate cancer should talk to their healthcare provider about the benefits and risks of the treatment, as well as the potential for side effects. They should also discuss their risk factors for side effects and how to manage them during and after treatment.

Immunotherapy

Immunotherapy is a type of cancer treatment that works by using the body's own immune system to fight cancer. It involves the use of drugs that target and activate the immune system to recognize and attack cancer cells.

In prostate cancer, immunotherapy may be used in advanced cases where other treatments have not been effective. There are several types of immunotherapy that may be used for prostate cancer, including checkpoint inhibitors, CAR T-cell therapy, and cancer vaccines.

Checkpoint inhibitors work by blocking proteins on the surface of immune cells that prevent them from attacking cancer cells. By blocking these proteins, checkpoint inhibitors can help the immune system recognize and attack cancer cells. CAR T-cell therapy involves modifying immune cells to better target cancer cells, while cancer vaccines work by stimulating the immune system to attack cancer cells.

Immunotherapy carries the risk of side effects, which can vary depending on the specific treatment used and the individual's response to treatment. Common side effects of immunotherapy for prostate cancer include:

Fatigue: Immunotherapy may cause fatigue and low energy levels.

Flu-like symptoms: Immunotherapy may cause symptoms such as fever, chills, and muscle aches.
Skin rash: Immunotherapy may cause a rash or other skin reactions.

Diarrhea: Immunotherapy may cause diarrhea or other digestive problems.

Men who are considering immunotherapy for prostate cancer should talk to their healthcare provider about the benefits and risks of the treatment, as well as the potential for side effects. They should also discuss their individual risk factors for side effects and how to manage them during and after treatment.

Clinical trials

Clinical trials are research studies that are designed to test new treatments, drugs, or medical procedures. In the context of prostate cancer, clinical trials are conducted to evaluate the effectiveness and safety of new therapies or to test combinations of existing treatments.

Participating in a clinical trial can offer several potential benefits for men with prostate cancer. It may provide access to new and potentially more effective treatments that are not yet widely available. It can also help researchers better understand the disease and improve treatments for future patients.

However, participating in a clinical trial also carries some risks. The new treatments being tested may not be effective, and may have unknown side effects. It is important for men considering participating in a clinical trial to understand the potential risks and benefits, and to discuss them with their healthcare provider.

Some clinical trials focus on treatments that are used after initial treatment has failed, while others are designed to test treatments that can be used in conjunction with standard therapies. In addition, some trials focus on improving the accuracy of diagnosis or the ability to predict a patient's response to treatment.

Men who are interested in participating in a clinical trial for prostate cancer should discuss their options with their healthcare provider. They can also find information about ongoing clinical trials by visiting clinicaltrials.gov or by contacting organizations that specialize in cancer research. It is important to carefully review the study protocols and requirements, and to understand what will be expected of the participant.

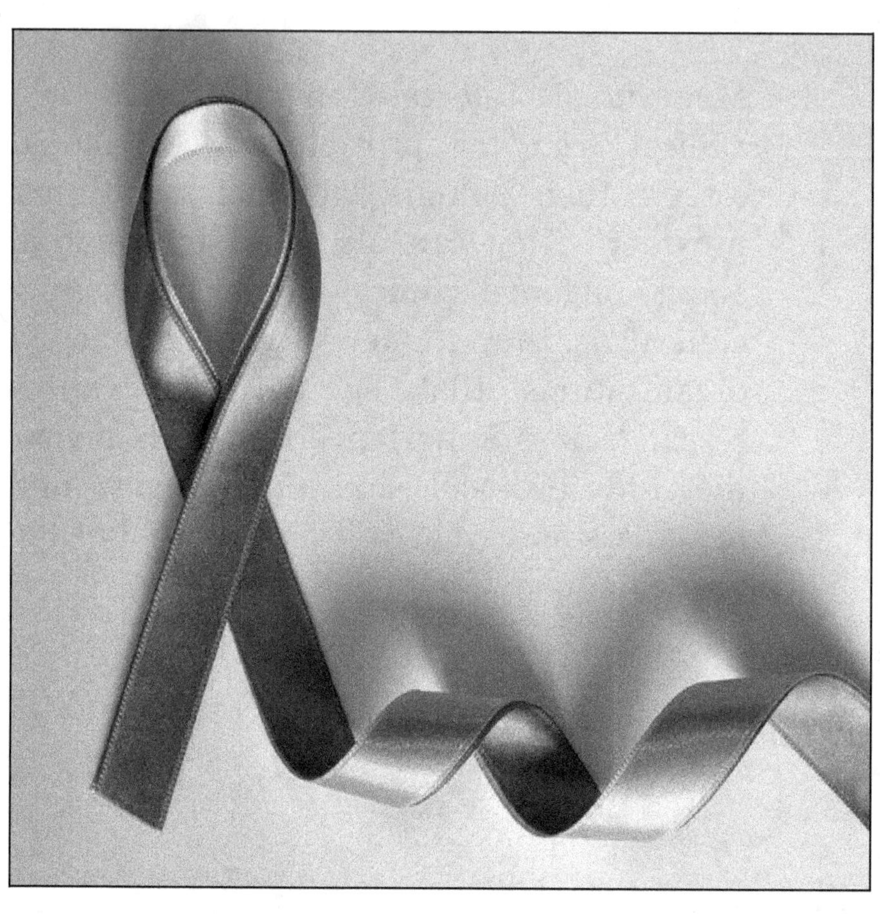

Chapter 3

Coping with Side Effects

Sexual Dysfunction

Sexual dysfunction is a common side effect of many prostate cancer treatments, including surgery, radiation therapy, hormone therapy, and chemotherapy. Coping with sexual dysfunction can be challenging, but there are strategies that men and their partners can use to manage these effects and maintain a satisfying sex life.

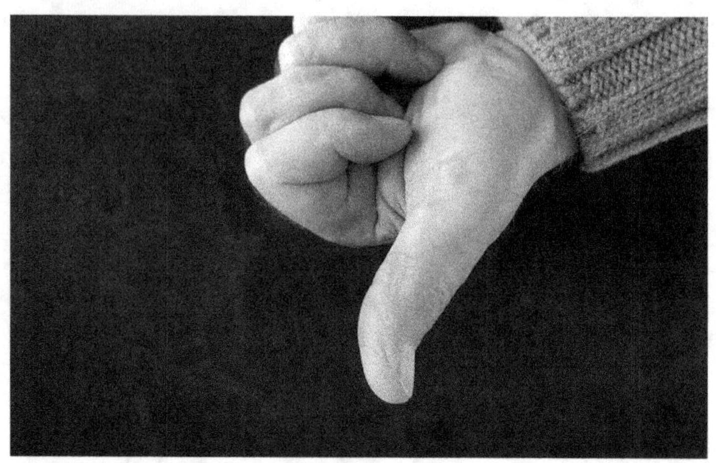

The first step in coping with sexual dysfunction is to talk to a healthcare provider about the specific side effects of the treatment being used. Healthcare providers can offer advice on coping strategies and may also be able to recommend medications or other treatments that can help.

In addition, men and their partners may find it helpful to work with a therapist or counselor who specializes in sexual health. These professionals can help couples explore alternative ways of expressing intimacy and sexuality, and may offer practical advice on managing sexual dysfunction.

Other strategies for coping with sexual dysfunction may include:

- Trying different sexual positions that are less physically demanding.
- Experimenting with different forms of intimacy, such as touching, kissing, and cuddling.
- Using aids such as vibrators, lubricants, or erectile dysfunction medications to help with sexual function.
- Maintaining a healthy diet and exercise routine to promote overall health and well-being.
- Joining a support group or online community for men and couples coping with sexual dysfunction.

It is important for men and their partners to communicate openly and honestly about their feelings and concerns related to sexual dysfunction. With the help of a healthcare provider and other professionals, many couples are able to manage sexual dysfunction and maintain a fulfilling sex life after prostate cancer treatment.

Urinary incontinence

Urinary incontinence is another common side effect of prostate cancer treatments, particularly after surgery. Incontinence can range from mild to severe, and can be temporary or long-lasting. Coping with urinary incontinence requires a combination of physical exercises, lifestyle changes, and practical strategies.

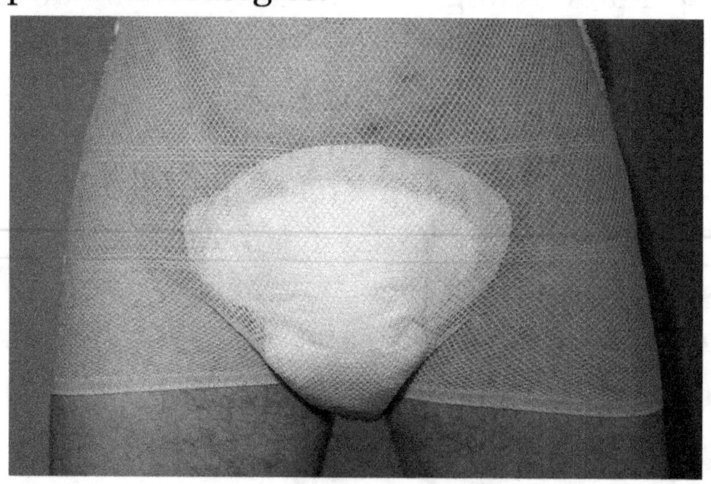

One of the most effective ways to manage urinary incontinence is through pelvic floor exercises, also known as Kegel exercises. These exercises involve contracting and releasing the muscles in the pelvic floor, which can help improve bladder control. Men can learn how to do these exercises from a healthcare provider, physical therapist, or through online resources.

In addition to pelvic floor exercises, men with urinary incontinence may find it helpful to:

- Avoid bladder irritants such as caffeine, alcohol, and spicy foods.
- Drink plenty of water and other fluids to stay hydrated.
- Go to the bathroom regularly, even if there is no urge to urinate.
- Use absorbent pads or undergarments to manage leaks.
- Wear loose-fitting clothing to avoid pressure on the bladder.

- Practice relaxation techniques such as deep breathing and meditation to reduce stress and anxiety.

If these strategies do not provide relief, there are medical interventions that can help manage urinary incontinence. These may include medication, bladder training, or surgical procedures.

It is important for men and their partners to communicate openly with their healthcare providers about any concerns related to urinary incontinence. With the right strategies and support, many men are able to manage this side effect and maintain a good quality of life after prostate cancer treatment.

Bowel problems

Bowel problems, such as diarrhea and constipation, are also common side effects of prostate cancer treatments. These side effects can be caused by radiation therapy, chemotherapy, and some medications used in hormone therapy. Coping with bowel problems may require a combination of lifestyle changes, medication, and dietary modifications.

If a man is experiencing diarrhea, it is important to stay hydrated and replenish lost fluids with water and electrolyte-rich beverages such as sports drinks or coconut water. Eating small, frequent meals and avoiding foods that can trigger diarrhea, such as high-fiber or spicy foods, may also help. In some cases, medication may be prescribed to slow the bowel movements.

If a man is experiencing constipation, increasing fiber intake through fruits, vegetables, and whole grains may help. Drinking plenty of water and engaging in regular physical activity may also promote regular bowel movements. In some cases, a healthcare provider may recommend a stool softener or laxative to help alleviate constipation.

It is important for men to communicate openly with their healthcare provider about any bowel problems they are experiencing. In some cases, adjusting the dosage or type of medication used in treatment may help alleviate these side effects. In addition, some men may benefit from seeing a registered dietitian to help develop a nutrition plan that can support bowel health during treatment.

Overall, coping with bowel problems requires patience and experimentation to find the strategies that work best for each individual. With the right support and guidance, men can manage these side effects and maintain a good quality of life during and after prostate cancer treatment.

Fatigue

Fatigue is another common side effect of prostate cancer treatment. It is often described as a feeling of extreme tiredness, weakness, or lack of energy that is not relieved by rest or sleep. Coping with fatigue can be challenging, but there are strategies that can help manage this side effect.

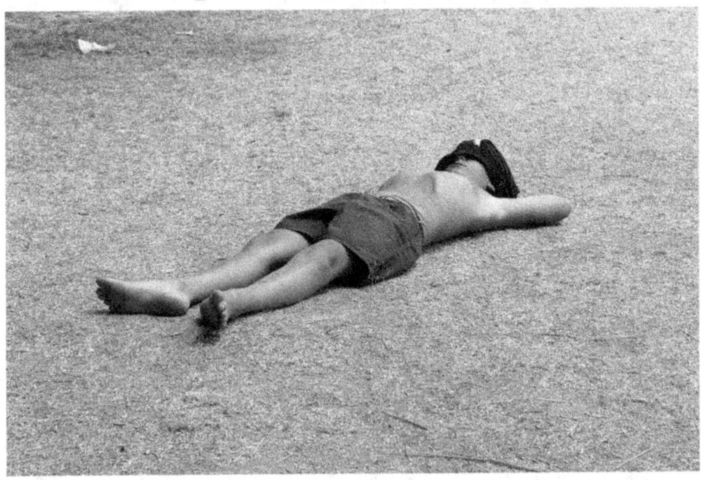

One of the most effective ways to manage fatigue is through regular physical activity. Exercise can help improve energy levels, reduce stress, and promote restful sleep. It is important for men to talk to their healthcare provider before starting an exercise program to ensure that it is safe and appropriate for their individual situation.

In addition to exercise, there are several other strategies that can help manage fatigue, including:

- Prioritizing rest and taking naps during the day as needed.
- Eating a balanced diet that includes plenty of whole foods, lean protein, and healthy fats.
- Staying hydrated by drinking plenty of water and other fluids throughout the day.
- Avoiding caffeine and alcohol, which can interfere with sleep and exacerbate fatigue.
- Practicing stress-reducing techniques such as deep breathing, meditation, or yoga.

- Accepting help from friends and family with daily tasks and responsibilities.
- Adjusting work schedules or taking time off as needed to rest and manage fatigue.

It is important for men to communicate openly with their healthcare provider about any concerns related to fatigue. In some cases, medication may be prescribed to manage fatigue, particularly if it is caused by anemia or other medical conditions. With the right strategies and support, many men are able to manage fatigue and maintain a good quality of life during and after prostate cancer treatment.

Emotional impact

Prostate cancer can have a significant emotional impact on men and their families. Receiving a cancer diagnosis can be a stressful and overwhelming experience, and many men may feel anxious, depressed, or fearful about the future. Coping with the emotional impact of prostate cancer can be as important as managing the physical side effects of treatment.

It is important for men to seek support from their healthcare team, family, and friends to manage the emotional impact of prostate cancer. Support groups and counseling services can also provide a safe space to share concerns and connect with others who are going through similar experiences.

Here are some strategies that can help manage the emotional impact of prostate cancer:

Education: Learn as much as possible about the diagnosis, treatment options, and potential side effects. Knowledge can help alleviate anxiety and empower men to make informed decisions about their care.

Self-care: Engage in activities that bring joy and relaxation, such as spending time in nature, reading, or listening to music. Taking care of oneself can help reduce stress and promote well-being.

Communication: Talk openly with loved ones about concerns and feelings related to the cancer diagnosis. This can help alleviate feelings of isolation and promote feelings of support and connection.

Mindfulness: Practice mindfulness techniques such as deep breathing or meditation to reduce stress and promote relaxation.

Professional support: Consider working with a mental health professional or joining a support group to receive additional emotional support and guidance.

Overall, managing the emotional impact of prostate cancer requires a combination of self-care, communication, and support from healthcare professionals, family, and friends. With the right strategies and support, men can cope with the emotional impact of prostate cancer and maintain a positive quality of life.

Chapter 4

Nutrition and Lifestyle Changes

Eating for prostate health

Eating a healthy diet is important for maintaining overall health and can be particularly beneficial for men with prostate cancer. There is evidence to suggest that certain dietary patterns may help prevent the development of prostate cancer or slow its progression. Here are some tips for eating for prostate health:

Eat a diet rich in fruits and vegetables: A diet that is rich in fruits and vegetables can help reduce the risk of prostate cancer. These foods are packed with vitamins, minerals, and antioxidants that can help protect against cancer.

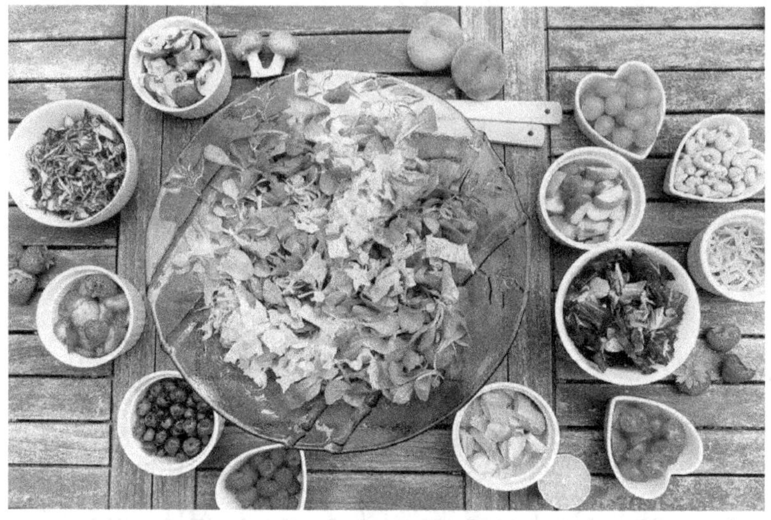

Choose whole grains: Whole grains are an excellent source of fiber, which is important for maintaining digestive health. Studies have also suggested that whole grains may help reduce the risk of prostate cancer.

Limit red meat and processed meats: There is evidence to suggest that consuming high amounts of red and processed meats may increase the risk of prostate cancer. It is recommended to limit these foods in the diet.

Include healthy fats: Consuming healthy fats, such as those found in nuts, seeds, and fatty fish, may help reduce the risk of prostate cancer. These foods are rich in omega-3 fatty acids, which have anti-inflammatory properties that can help protect against cancer.

Limit alcohol and caffeine: Alcohol and caffeine can irritate the bladder and contribute to urinary incontinence, a common side effect of prostate cancer treatment.

In addition to making dietary changes, there are several other lifestyle changes that men with prostate cancer can make to support their health, including:

Exercise regularly: Regular exercise can help reduce the risk of cancer and improve overall health. It is recommended to engage in moderate-intensity exercise for at least 150 minutes per week.

Maintain a healthy weight: Maintaining a healthy weight can help reduce the risk of prostate cancer and other chronic diseases.

Quit smoking: Smoking is a risk factor for many types of cancer, including prostate cancer. Quitting smoking can help reduce the risk of cancer and improve overall health.

Overall, making dietary and lifestyle changes can be an effective way for men with prostate cancer to support their overall health and well-being. It is important to consult with a healthcare provider before making significant changes to the diet or exercise routine.

Exercise and physical activity

Exercise and physical activity are important for maintaining overall health and can be particularly beneficial for men with prostate cancer. Regular exercise has been shown to improve physical function, reduce fatigue, improve quality of life, and potentially improve treatment outcomes for men with prostate cancer. Here are some tips for exercise and physical activity for men with prostate cancer:

Consult with a healthcare provider: Before starting any new exercise routine, it is important to consult with a healthcare provider. They can provide guidance on the types of exercises that are safe and appropriate for each individual.

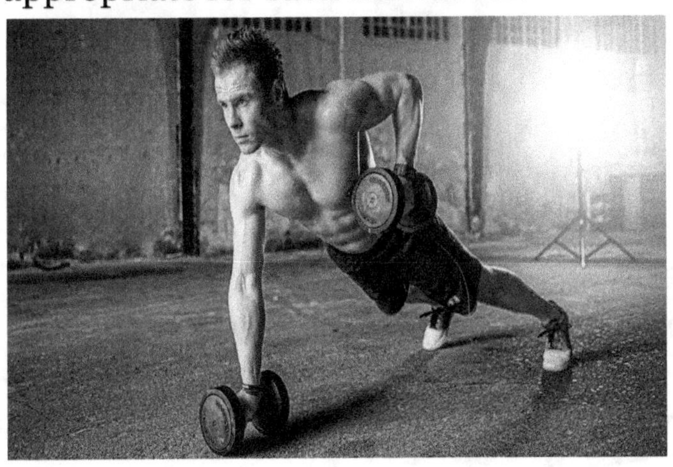

Choose a variety of exercises: A well-rounded exercise routine should include a variety of exercises, such as aerobic exercise, strength training, and flexibility exercises. Aerobic exercise, such as brisk walking or cycling, can improve cardiovascular health, while strength training can help build muscle and improve bone health. Flexibility exercises, such as yoga or stretching, can help improve range of motion and reduce the risk of injury.

Start slowly and gradually increase intensity: It is important to start slowly and gradually increase the intensity of exercise over time. This can help prevent injury and allow the body to adapt to the new activity level.

Incorporate physical activity into a daily routine: Simple changes such as taking the stairs instead of the elevator, walking or biking to work to run errands, or taking a walk after dinner can help increase physical activity levels.

Stay motivated: Exercise can be more enjoyable when done with others. Joining a fitness class or exercising with a friend can help keep motivation levels high.

In addition to exercise, other lifestyle factors such as sleep and stress management can also have an impact on overall health and well-being. Men with prostate cancer may benefit from incorporating stress-reducing techniques such as meditation, deep breathing, or yoga into their daily routines. Adequate sleep is also important for recovery and overall health.

Stress management

Stress management is an important component of a comprehensive approach to managing prostate cancer. Receiving a prostate cancer diagnosis can be a stressful and overwhelming experience, and stress can have a negative impact on physical and emotional well-being. Stress management techniques can help men with prostate cancer cope with the diagnosis, reduce anxiety, and improve their overall quality of life.

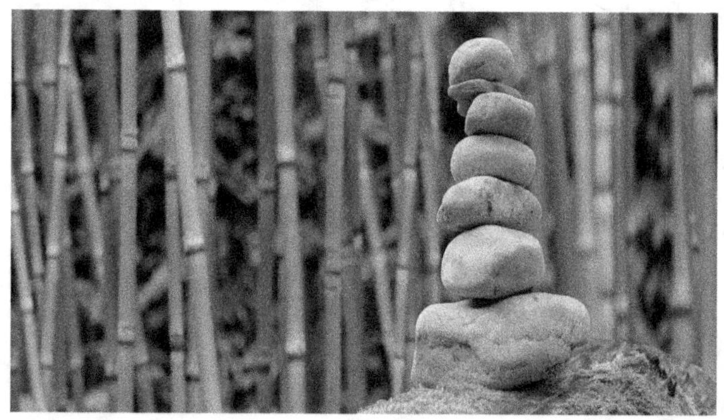

Here are some stress management techniques that may be helpful for men with prostate cancer:

Mindfulness meditation: Mindfulness meditation involves focusing on the present moment and becoming more aware of thoughts and feelings without judgment.

This can help reduce stress, anxiety, and depression, and improve overall well-being.

Deep breathing: Deep breathing exercises can help reduce stress and promote relaxation. One simple technique involves inhaling deeply through the nose, holding the breath for a few seconds, and exhaling slowly through the mouth.

Yoga: Yoga is a physical and spiritual practice that can help reduce stress, improve flexibility and strength, and promote overall well-being. There are many types of yoga, so it's important to find a practice that is appropriate for each individual.

Physical activity: Regular exercise can help reduce stress and improve overall well-being. This can include activities such as walking, jogging, swimming, or cycling.

Support groups: Joining a support group can help men with prostate cancer connect with others who are going through similar experiences. This can provide emotional support and help reduce feelings of isolation and anxiety.

Therapy: Therapy can be a helpful tool for managing stress and anxiety. A therapist can provide a safe and supportive environment to talk about feelings and develop coping strategies.

It's important for men with prostate cancer to find a stress management technique that works for them. Not all techniques work for everyone, so it may take some trial and error to find the best approach. Consulting with a healthcare provider or mental health professional can also provide guidance on effective stress management techniques.

Chapter 5

Support and Resources

Support groups and counseling services

A prostate cancer diagnosis can be a life-changing event and can cause a great deal of stress, anxiety, and depression. It's important for men with prostate cancer to have access to support and resources to help them cope with the emotional and practical challenges of the disease.

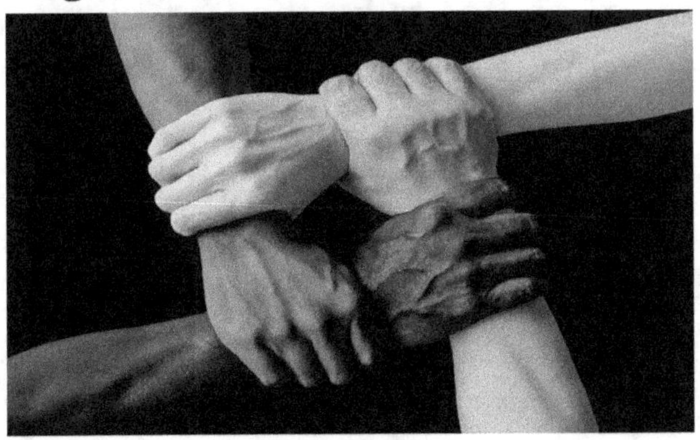

Here are some support and counseling resources for men with prostate cancer:

Support groups: Joining a support group can be a helpful way for men with prostate cancer to connect with others who are going through similar experiences. Support groups provide an opportunity to share feelings and experiences, receive emotional support, and gain practical information.

Counseling: Counseling can be a helpful tool for managing stress, anxiety, and depression. A mental health professional can provide a safe and supportive environment to talk about feelings and develop coping strategies.

National Cancer Institute (NCI): The NCI provides a variety of resources for men with prostate cancer and their families, including information about treatment options, support services, and clinical trials.

American Cancer Society (ACS): The ACS offers a wide range of services and resources for men with prostate cancer and their families, including a toll-free helpline, support groups, and educational materials.

Us TOO International: Us TOO International is a non-profit organization that provides support and educational resources for men with prostate cancer and their families. The organization offers a toll-free helpline, online support groups, and a range of educational materials.

Prostate Cancer Foundation (PCF): The PCF is a non-profit organization that funds research and provides educational resources for men with prostate cancer and their families. The organization offers a toll-free helpline, online support groups, and a range of educational materials.

It's important for men with prostate cancer to take advantage of the support and resources available to them. Talking with others who have gone through similar experiences can help reduce feelings of isolation and provide emotional support. Seeking professional counseling can also provide guidance and support in managing the emotional challenges of the disease.

Online resources and advocacy groups

In addition to the support and counseling resources mentioned earlier, there are also many online resources and advocacy groups that can provide valuable information and support for men with prostate cancer and their families. Here are a few examples:

ZERO - The End of Prostate Cancer: ZERO is a non-profit organization dedicated to ending prostate cancer. Their website provides information about treatment options, clinical trials, and support services.

They also offer an online support group and a toll-free helpline.

Malecare: Malecare is a non-profit organization that provides support and advocacy for men with prostate cancer. Their website includes information about treatment options, clinical trials, and support services. They also offer an online support group and a toll-free helpline.

Prostate Cancer Research Institute (PCRI): The PCRI is a non-profit organization that provides educational resources and support for men with prostate cancer and their families. Their website includes information about treatment options, clinical trials, and support services. They also offer a toll-free helpline.

Prostate Cancer Foundation (PCF): In addition to funding research, the PCF provides educational resources and support for men with prostate cancer and their families. Their website includes information about treatment options, clinical trials, and support services. They also offer an online support group and a toll-free helpline.

CancerCare: CancerCare is a non-profit organization that provides free counseling, support groups, and educational resources for people with cancer and their families. They offer a prostate cancer online support group and a toll-free helpline.

These online resources and advocacy groups can be a valuable source of information and support for men with prostate cancer and their families. They can help provide a sense of community, as well as valuable information about treatment options, clinical trials, and support services.

Financial assistance and insurance guidance

Dealing with a cancer diagnosis and its treatment can be overwhelming, and finances are often a significant concern. Here are some resources and guidance on financial assistance and insurance:

Cancer Financial Assistance Coalition (CFAC): CFAC is a coalition of organizations that provide financial assistance to cancer patients. They offer a searchable database of organizations that provide financial assistance for cancer-related expenses, such as transportation, lodging, and medication.

Patient Advocate Foundation (PAF): PAF provides case management services to help patients navigate the healthcare system, including insurance and financial issues. They offer assistance with insurance denials, appeals, and co-pay relief programs.

Social Security Administration (SSA): The SSA provides disability benefits for those who are unable to work due to their medical condition, including cancer. The SSA also offers the Compassionate Allowances program, which provides expedited processing of disability claims for certain conditions, including prostate cancer.

American Cancer Society (ACS): The ACS provides resources and guidance on managing the cost of cancer care. They offer information on insurance coverage, financial assistance programs, and tips for managing expenses.

Local Cancer Centers: Many cancer centers have financial counselors on staff who can provide guidance on insurance coverage and financial assistance options. It is essential to inquire with your treatment center about their financial assistance and counseling services.

It's essential to have an open conversation with your doctor, social worker, or hospital about the financial aspects of your treatment. They may be able to help you navigate the healthcare system and connect you with resources for financial assistance. Remember, you are not alone, and there are many resources available to help manage the financial burden of cancer treatment.

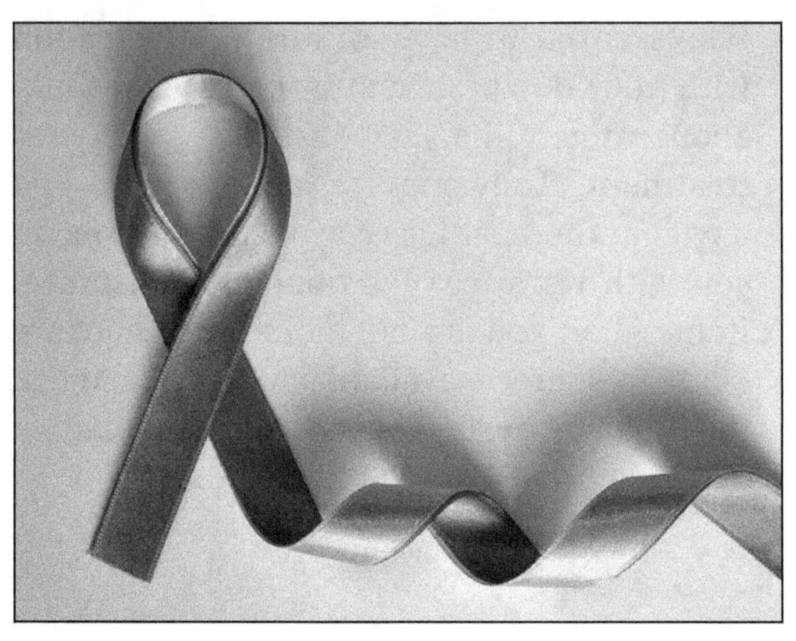

Chapter 6

Long-Term Management and Follow-Up

Post-treatment follow-up care

After treatment for prostate cancer, it's essential to continue with regular medical check-ups and follow-up care. Follow-up care is important to monitor for any signs of cancer recurrence or side effects from treatment. Here are some important considerations for post-treatment follow-up care:

Follow-up schedule: Your doctor will recommend a follow-up schedule based on your cancer stage, type of treatment, and other individual factors. Follow-up appointments will typically occur more frequently in the first few years after treatment and then become less frequent over time.

PSA tests: Prostate-specific antigen (PSA) tests are often used to monitor for cancer recurrence. A rise in PSA levels could be an indication of cancer recurrence or other prostate-related issues. PSA tests are typically performed at regular intervals following treatment.

Imaging tests: Imaging tests such as CT scans, bone scans, and MRIs may be used to monitor for cancer recurrence or progression.

Hormone therapy: For those who have undergone hormone therapy, regular monitoring of testosterone levels may be necessary to ensure that the cancer has not returned.

Managing side effects: It's important to continue to manage any ongoing side effects from treatment, such as sexual dysfunction or urinary incontinence. Your doctor can recommend strategies for managing these side effects or refer you to a specialist if necessary.

Healthy lifestyle: Maintaining a healthy lifestyle can help to reduce the risk of cancer recurrence and manage side effects. This includes regular exercise, a healthy diet, and stress management.

Communicating with your healthcare team: Keep an open line of communication with your healthcare team and report any changes in symptoms or side effects promptly.

In conclusion, post-treatment follow-up care is a critical aspect of prostate cancer management. By staying vigilant with follow-up appointments, PSA tests, and imaging tests, individuals can detect cancer recurrence early and receive timely treatment. It's also essential to continue to manage ongoing side effects from treatment and maintain a healthy lifestyle to reduce the risk of recurrence.

Monitoring for recurrence

Monitoring for prostate cancer recurrence is an important aspect of post-treatment follow-up care. Here are some of the ways that doctors monitor for recurrence:

PSA testing: Prostate-specific antigen (PSA) testing is commonly used to monitor for cancer recurrence after treatment. An increase in PSA levels can be a sign of cancer recurrence or residual cancer that was not completely removed during treatment. Typically, PSA levels are measured at regular intervals after treatment, with more frequent testing in the first few years after treatment.

Digital rectal exam (DRE): During a DRE, a doctor checks the prostate gland for any abnormalities or changes in size or shape that could be a sign of cancer recurrence.

Imaging tests: Imaging tests, such as CT scans, bone scans, and MRI, may be used to detect any cancer recurrence or spread to other parts of the body.

Biopsy: In some cases, a biopsy may be performed to confirm the presence of cancer recurrence. This is typically done when PSA levels rise or other symptoms suggest the possibility of cancer recurrence.

It's important to note that not all increases in PSA levels indicate cancer recurrence. Other factors, such as infection, inflammation, or an enlarged prostate, can also cause PSA levels to rise. Your doctor will consider all available information, including PSA levels, imaging tests, and physical exams, to determine whether further testing or treatment is necessary.

It's also important for individuals to report any new symptoms or changes in existing symptoms to their healthcare team promptly. Early detection of cancer recurrence can improve treatment outcomes and quality of life.

Living well after prostate cancer

Being diagnosed with prostate cancer can be a life-changing experience, but with proper care and support, many men can lead happy and healthy lives after treatment. Here are some tips for living well after prostate cancer:

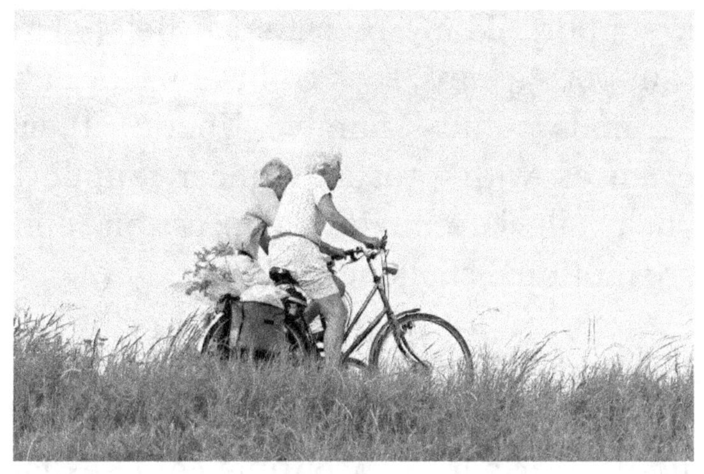

Maintain a healthy lifestyle: Eating a healthy diet, engaging in regular physical activity, and avoiding tobacco and excessive alcohol consumption can help promote overall health and reduce the risk of cancer recurrence.

Stay on top of follow-up care: Regular follow-up appointments and monitoring, including PSA testing and physical exams, can help detect any cancer recurrence or other health issues early, when treatment is more likely to be effective.

Seek support: Many men find it helpful to join support groups, seek counseling, or talk to friends and family about their experiences with prostate cancer. Support can help alleviate anxiety, depression, and other emotional challenges.

Address side effects: Treatment for prostate cancer can cause a range of side effects, including urinary incontinence, sexual dysfunction, fatigue, and bowel problems. It's important to work with your healthcare team to manage these side effects and address any concerns that may arise.

Manage stress: Prostate cancer can be a stressful experience, and stress can impact overall health and well-being. Finding ways to manage stress, such as through meditation, exercise, or hobbies, can be helpful for many men.

Consider participation in clinical trials: Clinical trials offer access to new and potentially more effective treatments for prostate cancer. Talk to your healthcare team about whether a clinical trial may be right for you.

Stay informed: Staying informed about prostate cancer research, treatment options, and resources can help you make informed decisions about your care and advocate for your own health.

In summary, living well after prostate cancer involves maintaining a healthy lifestyle, staying on top of follow-up care, seeking support, addressing side effects, managing stress, considering participation in clinical trials, and staying informed about the latest developments in prostate cancer research and treatment. With the right care and support, many men can lead happy and fulfilling lives after treatment for prostate cancer.

Conclusion

Encouragement and hope for prostate cancer survivors

Prostate cancer can be a challenging experience, but it's important to remember that there is hope for a bright future. With advances in medical treatments and ongoing research, more men are surviving and thriving after prostate cancer. It's important to stay informed, seek support, and prioritize self-care to promote overall health and well-being. By working closely with your healthcare team, managing side effects, and staying on top of follow-up care, you can feel empowered to live your best life after prostate cancer.

It's also important to recognize that every person's experience with prostate cancer is unique, and there is no "right" way to navigate this journey. Be kind to yourself and prioritize what works best for you and your health. With the right care, support, and mindset, you can look forward to a hopeful and fulfilling future as a prostate cancer survivor.

Call to action for awareness and advocacy

As we conclude this guide to surviving prostate cancer, it's important to recognize that awareness and advocacy are critical components of promoting better outcomes for prostate cancer patients and survivors. Prostate cancer affects many men and their families around the world, and it's important that we work together to raise awareness about the disease, its risk factors, and the importance of early detection and treatment.

One way to get involved is by supporting organizations that provide support, resources, and education to those affected by prostate cancer. These organizations can also play a critical role in funding research and advocacy efforts to advance the understanding and treatment of the disease.

Another way to get involved is by sharing your story and raising awareness in your own community. By talking openly and honestly about your experiences with prostate cancer, you can help reduce the stigma surrounding the disease and encourage others to prioritize their own health and well-being.

Remember, whether you are a prostate cancer survivor, caregiver, healthcare provider, or advocate, you have an important role to play in promoting awareness and advocating for better outcomes for those affected by the disease. Together, we can work towards a future where prostate cancer is detected early, treated effectively, and ultimately cured.

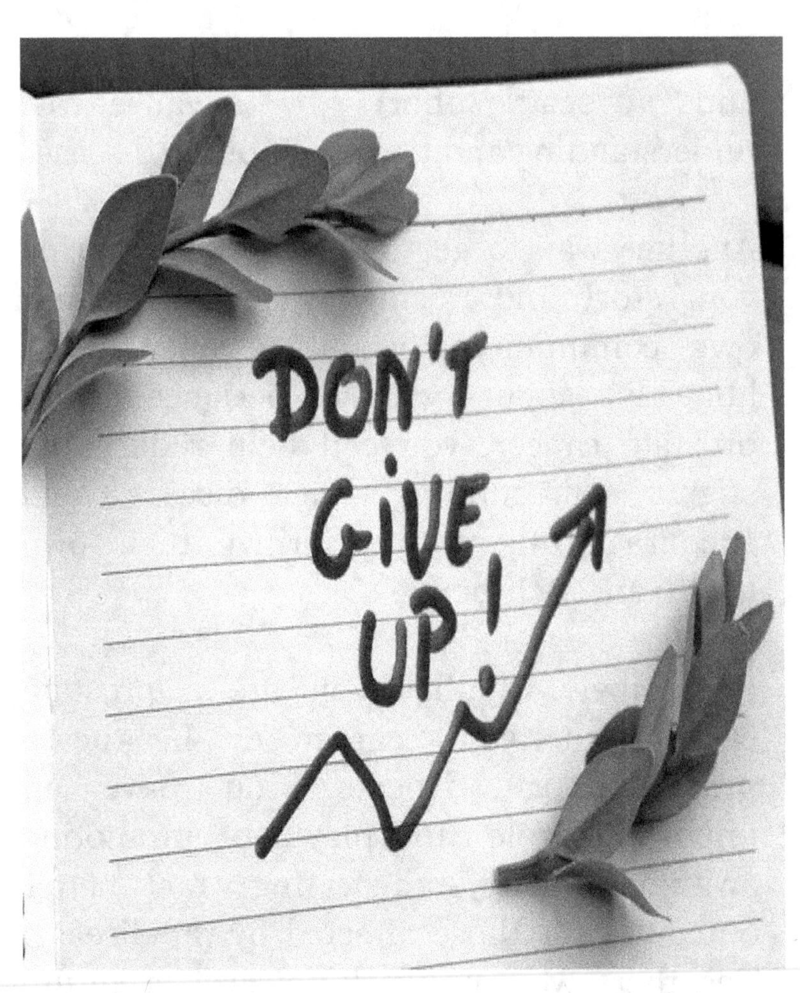
DON'T
GIVE
UP!